Gold Standard Management: The Key to High-Performance Hospitals

Your board, staff, or clients may also benefit from this book's insight. For more information on quantity discounts, contact the Health Administration Press Marketing Manager at (312) 424-9470.

This publication is intended to provide accurate and authoritative information in regard to the subject matter covered. It is sold, or otherwise provided, with the understanding that the publisher is not engaged in rendering professional services. If professional advice or other expert assistance is required, the services of a competent professional should be sought.

The statements and opinions contained in this book are strictly those of the author(s) and do not represent the official positions of the American College of Healthcare Executives or of the Foundation of the American College of Healthcare Executives.

Library of Congress Cataloging-in-Publication Data

Sherman, V. Clayton.
    Gold standard management : the key to high-performance hospitals / V. Clayton Sherman ; with Stephanie G. Sherman.
      p. ; cm.
    Includes bibliographical references.
    ISBN-13: 978-1-56793-286-7 (alk. paper)
    ISBN-10: 1-56793-286-X (alk. paper)
    1. Hospitals—United States—Administration. 2. Hospitals—United States—Personnel management. I. Sherman, Stephanie G. II. Title. [DNLM: 1. Hospital Administration—methods—United States. 2. Personnel Management—methods—United States. WX 150 S553g 2008]
    RA971.S4854 2008
    362.11068'3—dc22

                                                                                2007031403

The paper used in this publication meets the minimum requirements of American National Standard for Information Sciences—Permanence of Paper for Printed Library Materials, ANSI Z39.48-1984. ∞ ™

Acquisitions editor: Audrey Kaufman; Project manager: Amanda Bove; Layout editor: Chris Underdown; Cover designer: Chris Underdown

Health Administration Press
A division of the Foundation of the
    American College of Healthcare Executives
1 North Franklin Street, Suite 1700
Chicago, IL 60606-3529
(312) 424-2800

EDGE

CHAPTER 1

The New Opportunity to Excel

"If a man is called to be a street sweeper, he should sweep streets even as Michelangelo painted, or Beethoven composed music, or Shakespeare wrote poetry. He should sweep streets so well that all the host of heaven and earth will pause to say, here lived a great street sweeper who did his job well."

—The Rev. Dr. Martin Luther King, Jr.

When was the last time you encountered Michelangelo management—the management behind a delightful product or a smooth-as-silk organizational interaction? For many hospitals, operations fall short of art, poetry, or music. The discordant noise of less-than-the-best work systems and unhappy Customers and staff signals the need for change. This book guides rapid transformations in management. Though substantial efforts in healthcare have improved organization excellence and certain functions such as Customer service, a systemic method to move the entire management team to a standardized, high-level system of performance is missing. Talk of managing better is not new, and an active management prescription is for organizations to universally practice gold standard management in all functions (Khurana, Nohria, and Penrice 2005). ▶

WHAT IS GOLD STANDARD MANAGEMENT?

Gold standard management (GSM) is defined as

1. an edgy attitude and unrelenting commitment to the best;
2. a complete and thorough implementation of best-management practices in every department;
3. integration and unification of various management philosophies and schools of thought so that management is an integrated system rather than a group of independent components or disconnected programs;
4. specific management objectives and accountability that put work in the hands of competent people, give freedom to make change, expect results, use tough measures, and apply consequences; and
5. a requirement that all professional and technical staff implement their specialty's standards and best practices.

Using GSM, the management team eliminates management malpractice and violations of known best practices. Managers eradicate operational sludge and do not tolerate mediocrity.

Not Everything That Can Be Counted Counts

According to Einstein, "Not everything that can be counted counts, and not everything that counts can be counted." Terms like evidence-based management (Pfeffer and Sutton 2006) have gained popularity in healthcare. Evidence- or data-based decision making needs to occur whenever possible. However, situations occur where data are unavailable or arrive too late. What happens then?

The leader's job is not simply a logic exercise that compares data tables. In the absence of timely and appropriate data, managerial grist is individual judgment, values, and the ability to understand people's motivations. Evidence-based management is helpful as a component of GSM but is not always definitive or decisive by itself. According to Paul Glasziou, director of the Center for Evidence-Based Medicine in Oxford, England, "Some things can't be tested; some things are so obvious, they don't need it" (Gorman 2007).

Hospital leaders recognize the need to accept the truths in each

Figure 1.1—A Unified and Integrated Management Approach

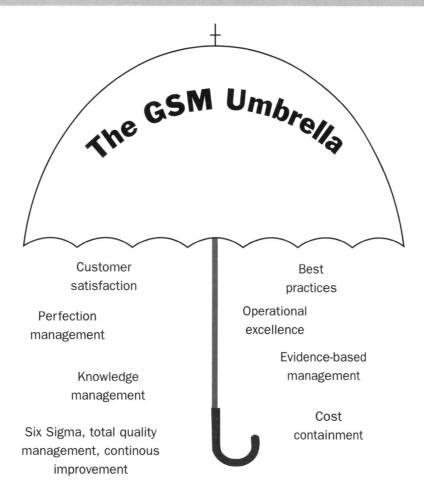

The GSM Umbrella

Customer
satisfaction

Best
practices

Perfection
management

Operational
excellence

Knowledge
management

Evidence-based
management

Six Sigma, total quality
management, continous
improvement

Cost
containment

component of professional management and the danger of accepting any one approach as the only approach. Because of multiple constituencies, time pressures, inadequate resources, and complex technologies, the modern hospital needs an eclectic, balanced management approach that ensures high-quality outcomes at the best possible cost and provides a high degree of satisfaction for Customers and staff. Figure 1.1 shows how GSM unifies the various components of professional management.

The New Partnership: Gold Standard Management and Gold Standard Medicine

The practice of medicine in the United States is moving rapidly toward evidence-based, standardized, and defined clinical protocols. The reasons are many, but in sum the driver is expanded knowledge that leads to best practices—the gold standard. Medical knowledge increases every year. The old saying that medical practice is both a science and an art is giving way to demands for more science and less art. Although feelings, intuitions, and judgments are part of human decision making, they are often a poor substitute for best practices.

To that end, the Institute of Medicine and other policy groups are recommending that Congress cut Medicare physician payments and use a portion of the savings to fund rewards to physicians who demonstrate high-quality, patient-centered, and efficient healthcare (Pear 2006). The drive for gold standard medicine is on, and that calls for a new management response in healthcare management. Best practices in healthcare delivery can only be delivered when teamed with best practices in management.

The era of gold standard healthcare has arrived, and both medicine and management face a win-win opportunity. When the new wave of medical thinking encounters resistance from the physician community, management needs to insist that all physicians who are granted privileges practice only gold standard medicine. In like fashion, when management battles to install GSM, physician demands for better support systems, staff training, Customer relationship training, and just-in-time systems can push management's change agenda forward.

A natural alliance is forming among new breed leaders (the young managers and physicians who represent the future). This younger generation clearly sees that it is in their mutual professional interest to support each other's agendas. Physicians should expect gold standard *management* and executives should expect gold standard *medicine* to deliver gold standard care (see Figure 1.2). Only in tight alignment can organizational results and best clinical outcomes be simultaneously achieved.

Figure 1.2—Collaboration Creates Gold Standard Outcomes

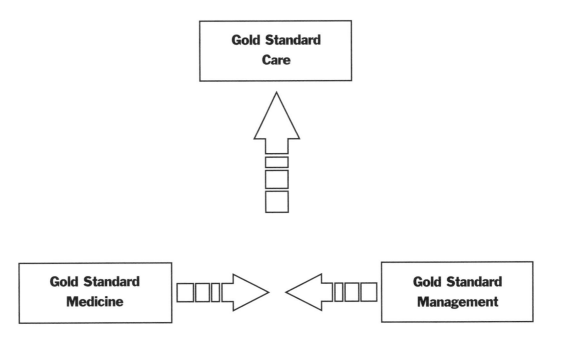

Heavy civil and criminal charges are being pressed against those who practice less-than-the-best medicine. An interesting legal development that aids good science is the increased legal defensibility of physicians who follow endorsed gold standard clinical protocols and the punishments of physicians whose procedures are outside gold standard clinical protocols (Leahy 1989).

Consequences will apply to physicians who do not practice medicine according to the gold standard.

Less-than-the-best management complicates and delays the movement toward gold standard medicine. A key illustration is the slow implementation of information technology (IT) in U.S. hospitals. Well entrenched in other industries for 20 years, data management's slow and uneven adoption in healthcare is now devastatingly highlighted in research from the Institute of Medicine (Gesensway 2004). The Leapfrog Group (2007), speaking for many of the nation's largest employers, has made IT its number-one demand in an expression of justifiable impatience.

THE STANDARDS REVOLUTION

Many of the world's best organizations are now operating by the rules of strategic standardization. The concept is powerful, and evidence of its power is growing. (Sherman 1999). There are two primary parts to the strategy:

1. *Standards.* Best-in-class standards represent a combination of best cost, highest-quality outcomes, and the most Customer-satisfying healthcare experiences. Best standards represent the path to product/service differentiation and competitive advantage. Organizations that pursue best-in-class standards of performance win.
2. *Standardization.* Standardization of best practices, technology,

people's skill levels, and methods is the second input required to build a system. This yields tremendous cost advantages, speed, and ease of operation. A lack of standardization means that most U.S. hospital chains are not systems, regardless of their marketing language. However, they have the potential to become true systems by employing standardization, thereby achieving extraordinary performance improvement.

The Standards Opportunity

Effective executives know that the standard is to meet at least the hospital industry's benchmark and preferably higher. Executives should position their organization somewhere between the best in the industry and the best in the world. This is the safest position to be in because operating at any lower level assumes the greatest risk of failure. Figure 1.3 shows how business performance improves with elevated standards.

The higher management sets organization performance standards, the more powerful its business outcomes and the greater its advantages against competitors. A recent study of Medicare data confirms this:

Rx FOR SUCCESS

Have a meeting between physicians and executives to gain support for a gold standard care initiative that includes both medical and management practices.

The top 5% of U.S. hospitals are pulling away from the pack in terms of improvements in risk-adjusted patient mortality and complication rates from the period of 2002 to 2004. Patients undergoing common inpatient procedures at the best hospitals had a 27% lower average risk of dying in the hospital and a 14% lower risk of complications than at other hospitals, based on an analysis of Medicare data.... Across the 26 conditions studied...if all Medicare patients had been treated comparably to the treatment patients received at the best 5% of hospitals, "152,966 lives may have been saved and 21,896 patients may have avoided a major postoperative complication" (*Modern Healthcare* 2006).

Figure 1.3—Business Performance Improves With Elevated Standards

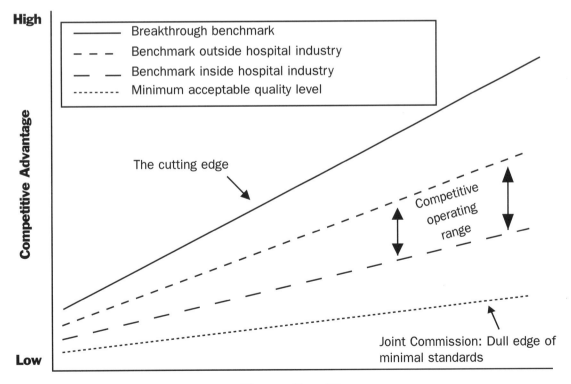

As the gap between the average organization's performance and the best hospital's performance widens, chances to remain competitive or survive decline.

The Standardization Moment

Executives are at a moment when they can pursue standardization. The following objectives should be high on every executive's operational to-do list:

1. Develop the IT backbone necessary to assist universal electronic patient records and the seamless digital flow of information between departments, physicians, and agencies.
2. Reduce variance in the number and types of supplies and equipment by having fewer suppliers with tighter performance and efficiency targets.
3. Streamline pharmacy services with the overall goal of having fewer suppliers, fewer drug variations, lower costs, and tighter controls.
4. Pursue lower costs and pricing targets—a truly unmet need and therefore an opportunity for dominance.
5. Implement best practices for staffing with a focus on low turnover, high skill levels, and esprit de corps among staff and physicians.

BENEFITS OF GOLD STANDARD MANAGEMENT

Benefits of GSM are substantial, immediate, and predictable. Organizations willing to do the work of installing GSM could achieve the following outcomes:

1. Increased Customer satisfaction ratings
2. Significant cost savings in the first year and a sustained, healthy economic performance with substantial improvements on cost and quality targets
3. A specific model that gives hardworking but results-poor leaders a method to make significant improvements in profitability, Customer satisfaction, Associate satisfaction, and work and quality processes
4. Managers who are on the same page and show people how to work together to achieve the highest levels of performance
5. Rapid dominance in competitive markets

Goshen Health System in Goshen, Indiana, implemented GSM beginning in 1998. Since then, they have achieved the following (Dague 2006):

THE MOM TEST

Would your mom approve of the management of your shop? If not, it is probably not gold standard.

- The lowest turnover in the state (nursing turnover at 1.25 percent in 2005 and 2006, down from a beginning rate of 27 percent)
- Press Ganey Summit Award for patient satisfaction ratings in the 95th percentile in 2004, 2005, and 2006
- Designation as a multiyear magnet hospital
- Profits of $11 million in 2006 after starting in 1988 with three weeks of cash
- Morale scores at 97th percentile as measured by HR Solutions International, Inc.
- No layoffs

Such achievements are possible at your hospital and are typical when following a GSM approach.

QUESTIONS FOR THE LEADER

1. As a leader, are you ready to make the move to GSM? Can you energize your management team around this opportunity?
2. Can you collaborate with the clinical leadership of your organization to form a strategic alliance that favors both gold standard medicine and management?

NOTE

1. The words Customer and Associate (employee) are capitalized to stress the importance of these central groups. Many healthcare organizations are now following this convention as well. Think of it this way: Capitalizing these words is a no-cost way to communicate something very valuable to these audiences and to keep our own thinking straight.

REFERENCES

Dague, J. O. 2006. E-mail communication with the author, July 5.

Gesensway, D. 2004. "The Case for Computerizing Health Care Now, Not Later." American College of Physicians *Observer*, April. [Online information; retrieved 1/12/07.] http://www.acponline.org/journals/news/apr04/computer.htm.

Gorman, C. 2007. "Are Doctors Just Playing Hunches?" *Time*, February 26, 52–54. [Online article; retrieved 6/1/07.] http://www.time.com/time/magazine/article/0,9171,1590448,00.html.

Khurana, R., N. Nohria, and D. Penrice. 2005. "Is Business Management a Profession?" *Harvard Business School Working Knowledge*. [Online article; retrieved 2/1/06.] http://hbswk.hbs.edu/item/4650.html.

Leahy, R. E. 1989. "Rational Health Policy and the Legal Standard of Care: A Call for Judicial Deference to Medical Practice Guidelines." *California Law Review* 77 (6): 1483–1528.

Leapfrog Group. 2007. "What Does Leapfrog Ask Hospitals?" [Online information; retrieved 6/1/07.] http://www.leapfroggroup.org/for_consumers/hospitals_asked_what.

Modern Healthcare. 2006. "Top Hospitals Continue to Improve Faster." *Modern Healthcare* Online. [Online Information; retrieved 2/6/06.] http://www.modernhealthcare.com.

Pear, R. 2006. "Medicare Links Doctors' Pay to Practices." *The New York Times*, December 2. [Online article; retrieved 6/1/07.] http://www.nytimes.com/2006/12/12/washington/12health.html?ex = 1323579600&en = 15492d7300975ccb&ei = 5088&partner = rssnyt&emc = rss.

Pfeffer, J., and R. Sutton. 2006. "Evidence-Based Management." *Harvard Business Review* 84 (1): 63–74.

Sherman, V. C. 1999. *Raising Standards in American Healthcare: Best People, Best Practices, Best Results*. San Francisco: Jossey-Bass.

CHAPTER 2

Deconstruction and Reinvention

"A house pulled down is half rebuilt."

—Proverb

To gain edge, speed, and robustness, your organization must lose dullness, slowness, and apathy. Part of the task of sharpening performance in your organization is to remove the aspects that slow performance. This work is preliminary to any effort to create a GSM environment.

Organizations discover that breakout performance is only possible after they break through the logjam of reasons why "it will not work here." An analogy to building a house is helpful: Before the foundation can be poured, the site must be cleared. Clearing the site, or deconstructing old ways of thinking, is a necessary step prior to installing GSM. ▶

THE DECONSTRUCTION REQUIREMENT

Criticism of the healthcare industry is valid when it is from corporate leaders who understand the management game. The rise of the Leapfrog Group and business groups such as the National Business Coalition on Health signals the greater management community's intense dissatisfaction with how healthcare is managed and their intentions to support only providers who increase their standards of performance.

The GSM challenge is to create a leadership culture that aggressively seeks new methods and best practices so that skills are systematically upgraded.

Build a Culture of Creative Destruction

Executives need to endorse an atmosphere that creates new approaches to doing work and removes old, less efficient ways. Imagine that you are frustrated with encountering too many reasons why things could not be streamlined, and you create a bounty system: $50 for every improved form, $100 for killing an unneeded report, $500 for committees that could put themselves out of existence. Old clutter will quickly fade away.

An organization cannot embrace its future by carrying the dead weight of its past while installing new processes. Executives should find something bureaucratic to execute—something to kill, maim, or amputate—and do it systematically and frequently.

Targets of Deconstruction

Targets to deconstruct prior to launching GSM include the following:

1. *Managers.* Remove managers who have given ample evidence of their inadequate performance and who have not improved. Do not make the common mistake of thinking that managers with poor performance need more training (Sherman 1987).
2. *Committees.* Reduce the number of committees, meetings, participants, and hours per meeting.
3. *Conflict.* Interdepartmental conflicts require staff swaps—make teams who are in conflict swap responsibilities by working a shift or two in the other department. Then, have them sit down and find a solution to prevent conflict from becoming a recurring issue.

Form the management team into small groups. Give the groups one hour to create lists of factors that hamper their ability to perform. Once the management team identifies the factors, ask the following questions:

- What slows down our management work?
- When is freedom to act inadequate?
- Where is information, communication, or training needed?
- Where are resources unnecessarily difficult to obtain?
- Where is timeliness of executive or organizational response an issue?
- What tools would improve management work?

4. *Negative energy.* Conversations that address problems and do not generate solutions create negative energy. Create a "no negative energy" rule: If you do not have an alternative solution, do not talk about the problem.

5. *Drift.* Set 30-day deadlines on all assigned projects. Executives must give approvals in seven days. Push work forward by not letting it pile up.

6. *Bureaucratic drag.* Require no more than two signatures on a requisition. If a requisition takes three signatures, then someone involved is not necessary.

7. *Performance expectations.* Declare a new set of performance expectations from managers. Use the Leader's Credo presented in the appendix.

Think about what other targets you could add to this list. A tremendous amount of work going on in your organization is not necessary. You do not get paid for work, only for results.

SCHEDULED REINVENTION

All processes, products, and policies obsolesce and degrade through time. Edgy organizations are quick and systematic in their approach to renewal; they toss out the old before the old slows them down. A home owner either can make repairs and improvements early in the maintenance schedule or can wait until the current condition has deteriorated. Many hospitals are way behind in repairs, replacements, renewals, and rehabilitation. This is particularly crippling when it comes to management policies and procedures.

Top-Down Reinvention

Figure 2.1 provides a schedule of systematic renewal of policies and management practices and ensures that each work element has a point on the calendar for review. Beware of superficial reviews that only condone what is already in place. Set an expectation that 25 percent of all policy and procedures are materially changed and improved each year rather than merely updated; this ensures that your organization is dumping the old. Once top management has this in place, cascade the concept down into each team.

Reinventing the Managerial Milieu

Nothing dulls an organization's edge as much as malpractice in management:

Figure 2.1—Scheduled Reinvention: A Top Management Calendaring Scheme

Month	Work Arena
1	Redefine mission: vision, values, and goals
2	Update strategic and marketing plans
3	Key result area groups identify key initiatives and write tactical plans
	Quarter's organization emphasis: best people

Month	Work Arena
4	Identify organization resource budget—do not let money dictate dreams
5	Revisit organization structure and human resources plan
6	Retune communications and socialization
	Quarter's organization emphasis: high satisfaction

Month	Work Arena
7	Training and organization learning
8	Retune information systems, revise measures, and increase accountability
9	Reward, recognition, and celebration systems review
	Quarter's organization emphasis: high quality

Month	Work Arena
10	Annual plan for department work/budget/people growth
11	Departments proceed to quarterly work plans
12	Audit organization and management processes and outcomes
	Quarter's organization emphasis: low cost

The troublesome fact is that mediocre management is the norm. This is not because some people are born without the management gene or because the wrong people get promoted or because the system can be manipulated—although all these things happen all the time. The overwhelmingly most common explanation is much simpler: capable management is so extraordinarily difficult that few people look good no matter how hard they try. Most of those lackluster managers we all complain about are doing their *best* to manage well (Teal 1996, 35).

More accurately, most managers are doing the best they know how to do, not the best they could do. Healthcare organizations do not need new managers as much as current managers need new skill development and a new managerial milieu.

IS HEALTHCARE MANAGEMENT A PROFESSION?

A debate currently raging in the American management community is whether management is a true profession or merely a trade (Khurana, Nohria, and Penrice 2005). Many people in management, across all industries, view themselves as tradespeople. They occupy seats of authority, put in their time, drink coffee, and eat doughnuts in the cafeteria, but they do not have skills to do the necessary tasks.

Vince Lombardi once famously observed, "Show me a good loser, and I'll show you a loser." Many people struggling to make healthcare work are not losers, but many are ineffective and unsuccessful. Why do these healthcare managers and management teams come up short? The answer is that they are unprepared amateurs. Even if positively motivated, they are not in the ranks of professionals.

GSM begins with gold standard managers. They thrive in an environment where excellence is expected and delivered on a daily basis—indeed, they become the yardsticks of quality. The winning organization knows that careful selection and grooming of this cadre spells its future.

QUESTIONS FOR THE LEADER

1. What targets would you pick in a deconstruction effort?
2. Do you think your management team would embrace a leader's credo? If they have no interest in commitment, what should you do?
3. How will you emphasize or celebrate the creative aspect of removing old ways of doing things

REFERENCES

Khurana, R., N. Nohria, and D. Penrice. 2005. "Is Business Management a Profession?" *Harvard Business School Working Knowledge.* [Online article; retrieved 2/1/06.] http://hbswk.hbs.edu/item/4650.html.

Sherman, V. C. 1987. *From Losers to Winners: How to Manage Problem Employees and What to Do If You Can't*. New York: American Management Association.

Teal, T. 1996. "The Human Side of Management." *Harvard Business Review* 74 (6): 35–44.

CHAPTER 3

Organization

Firepower and Targets

"The secret of all victory lies in the organization of the non-obvious."

—Oswald Spengler

Management must provide two fundamentals that serve as a platform or infrastructure for future organization achievement. First, management must create a new American hospital—the kind of organization that allows people to produce results. Second, management must define targets that really matter—those that are beneficial to the organization and that motivate the people who do the work.

A MODEL FOR A HIGH-PERFORMANCE HOSPITAL

Sometimes it seems that the only things that evolve naturally in an organization are friction, disorder, and poor performance. Organizational dysfunctionality is the quagmire for good intentions. The old hospital model suffered from silo thinking, was overlaid with countless do-little committees, segregated occupational groups, and underemphasized the importance of training and recognition for the organization's people. ▸

Proper execution of GSM creates a new model for high-performance hospitals. The new model functions more efficiently and provides a more personal work environment than experienced in most healthcare organizations. Also, the new model is congruent with current research on what really works in creating high-performance organizations (Nohria, Joyce, and Robertson 2003). A high-performance hospital is possible only when the following elements are in place:

- Uncommon leadership
- Values-driven performance
- Associate-powered work environment
- Quality-controlled work systems
- Customer-focused processes
- Future-focused financial and market strategies

Organization Success Ingredients

Figure 3.1 shows the major elements in play within a high-performance hospital. At the center are the groups of players involved in healthcare delivery: the Customer, the Associate, and the Leader. The Customer receives service/care from the Associate—this is what the business is all about. Leaders support and serve this transaction, and they are subordinate to it as they monitor and enhance its outcomes. The work of GSM transformation is to install best practices in each of the areas shown in Figure 3.1.

UNCOMMON LEADERSHIP. Everything begins with leadership, and the performance cycle begins here. A new leadership model is necessary before the work of GSM can go forward. The primary task of the leader is to grow the skills, attitudes, and performance of the people, the organization's prime competitive advantage. The second priority for leadership is improving work systems. One way to articulate leadership's job is to see that leaders exist to mold the organization to fit what Customers need and what Associates require. Effective leaders spend a great deal of time listening to Customers and Associates, believing what they say, and then doing what is called for.

VALUES-DRIVEN PERFORMANCE. High-performance hospitals are *not* market driven; they are values driven. One of the values of a high-performance hospital is Customer satisfaction, whereby leaders choose to *serve* the market, not be *driven*

WORDS OF WISDOM

The people who are doing the work are the moving force.... My job is to create a space for them, to clear out the rest of the organization, and keep it at bay.

—Steve Jobs, CEO of Apple, Inc.

by it. High-performance hospitals eradicate and replace repressive elements with job joy and satisfaction in creative work, where ideas are born and problems overcome.

GSM leaders create work conditions that allow the people at work to develop and achieve greatness. As the work environment evolves to a "family feel," which senior workers often report has been lost, the hospital is increasingly able to move quickly to solve problems and reduce barriers. In this environment, it becomes possible for people to develop and produce at their best.

ASSOCIATE-POWERED WORK ENVIRONMENT. Associates are focused on two targets: (1) satisfy their Customers

Figure 3.1—The New American Hospital

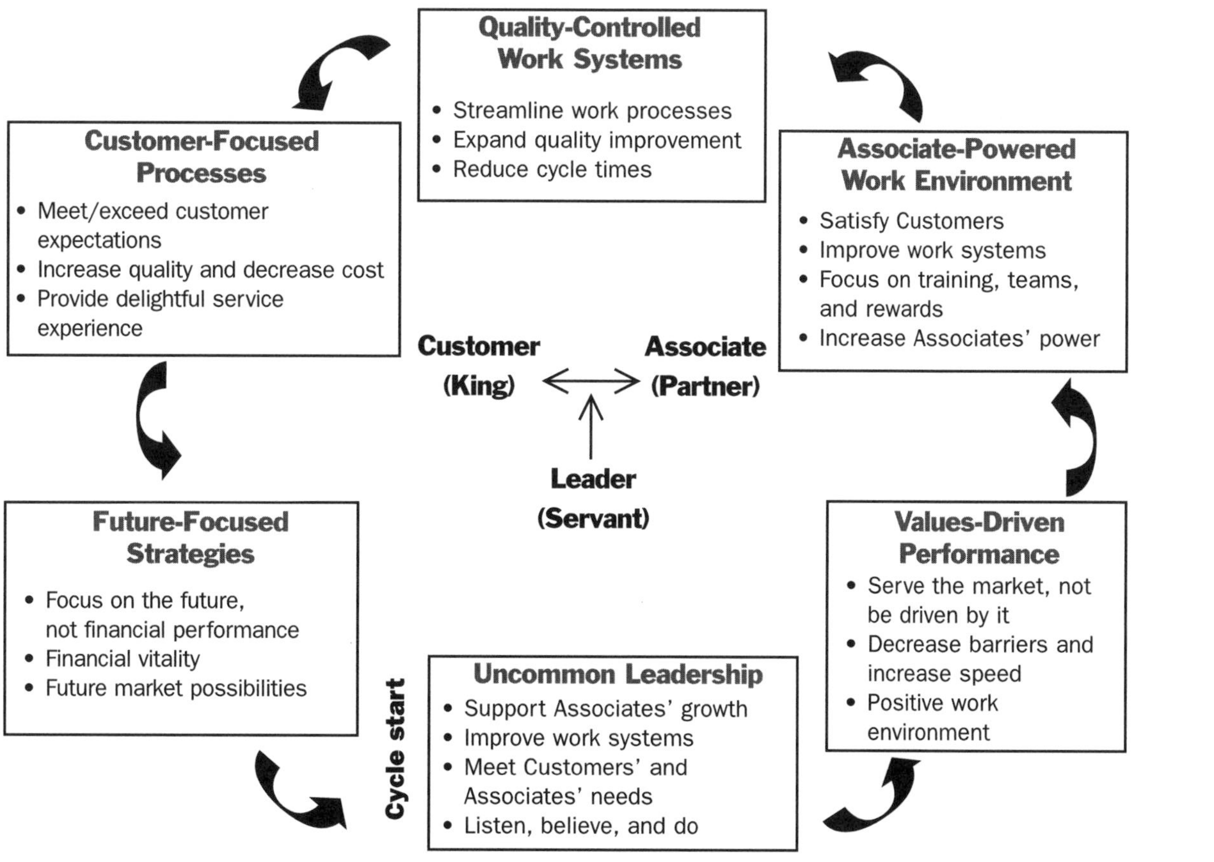

Quality-Controlled Work Systems
• Streamline work processes
• Expand quality improvement
• Reduce cycle times
Customer-Focused Processes
• Meet/exceed customer expectations
• Increase quality and decrease cost
• Provide delightful service experience
Associate-Powered Work Environment
• Satisfy Customers
• Improve work systems
• Focus on training, teams, and rewards
• Increase Associates' power
Customer (King)
Associate (Partner)
Leader (Servant)
Future-Focused Strategies
• Focus on the future, not financial performance
• Financial vitality
• Future market possibilities
Values-Driven Performance
• Serve the market, not be driven by it
• Decrease barriers and increase speed
• Positive work environment
Cycle start
Uncommon Leadership
• Support Associates' growth
• Improve work systems
• Meet Customers' and Associates' needs
• Listen, believe, and do

and (2) improve the work system. The strategy is to build a smarter and more capable work team through providing enriched and bigger jobs, more training (an investment with immediate high return), less restrictive supervision, cross-functional teams, and a greater emphasis on recognition and rewards. The power of releasing Associates' intellectual capital fuels competitive advantage. People do not need to be empowered, because they already have the power. Leadership needs to stop de-powering them and to get out of their way.

QUALITY-CONTROLLED WORK SYSTEMS.
This area focuses on tasks and projects needed to streamline work processes. On this to-do list are tasks of reengineering, expanding continuous quality improvement, improving IT, reducing cycle times, and standardizing clinical and infrastructure processes. In the work systems and processes, the hospital creates something valued by the market—quality care at affordable prices. This is impossible to achieve if previous steps have been short-changed.

CUSTOMER-FOCUSED PROCESSES. A Customer is the beneficiary of work done by each jobholder. This downstream orientation determines not only how well present tasks are done, but also whether Customer expectations are being met or exceeded. The Customer's primary wants are for more consistent quality outcomes, lower costs, and a delightful service experience. The task is clear: Install changes necessary to achieve these targets, beginning with a long list of Customer irritations that need to be removed and an equally long list of low-cost or no-cost items that add value, pleasure, and convenience to the Customer experience.

FUTURE-FOCUSED FINANCIAL AND MARKET STRATEGIES. Both profit and revenue growths are natural outcomes of a high-performance hospital. Whereas many hospitals are preoccupied with financial performance, GSM leadership knows that the focus is upstream. When leadership attends to the previous five factors of uncommon leadership, values-driven performance, Associate-powered work environment, quality-controlled work systems, and Customer-focused processes, financial vitality and future market possibilities are a natural consequence.

Results of the Model

Competing management philosophies and practices currently at work in the hospital industry are unlikely to succeed and do not share an equal track record of success. An organization running on GSM fuel is built for speed of response and high adaptability to massive change. It is fast, flexible, fun, and robust. Most importantly, such hospitals are competitively dominant. In some form, the high-performance hospital is what most healthcare organizations must become if they are to survive.

COMPETITIVELY DOMINANT. Many executives have spent too much time worrying about external issues, like competition and regulatory problems, and have spent too much time away from their organizations in various political and lobbying efforts. Effective leaders realize that the secret is to focus on the variables internal to the organization, most of which are controllable and produce results that are far more powerful.

DEFINING TARGETS THAT REALLY MATTER

It has been said that America's consistent problem is "putting second things first." Healthcare leaders need to determine which targets matter. Effective leaders know that goals that only clone what competitors are doing are a sure way to doom the organization. High-performing hospitals and their leaders need to define targets that really matter to the hospital.

What Matters to People?

Many people are not excited about going to work. Research shows that only 50 percent of Associates are satisfied with their jobs, 66 percent do not identify with their employer's business goals, and 25 percent are only "showing up to collect a paycheck" (Conference Board 2005). Something is clearly missing. The missing piece is a feeling among individual staff that they are engaged in something meaningful.

Small goals and incremental changes do not motivate people. President Reagan (1981) said it well: America is "too great a nation to limit ourselves with small dreams." Indeed, would you recommend for hire an executive who did not want to be best in class? Asking people to strive for excellence is not burdensome; rather, it is motivating and inspiring. The person with big dreams is more powerful than the one with all the facts.

GSM uses big, hairy, audacious goals (BHAGs) (Collins 2001) to make work exciting, and it creates the kind of organization that makes attaining those targets possible.

What Matters to the Business?

Vince Lombardi, once challenged with the notion that the important thing in sports was the playing, not the winning, responded, "If winning isn't everything, why do they keep score?" Effective leaders must measure achievement. It was not that long ago that Customer satisfaction was not measured, a classic symptom of activity divorced from purpose.

The balanced scorecard (Kaplan and Norton 1996) has become a standard tool in management, and it is part of the GSM approach. A study by Rigby and Bilodeau (2007) reported that 66 percent of global corporations are using a balanced scorecard, only a decade after its introduction. Correctly used, balanced scorecards can be a powerful force in driving change. However, many hospital leaders still do not use the tool well. When misapplied, it can waste time, be

confusing, and substantiate mediocrity of organizational performance.

In practice, people customize the balanced scorecard to suit their environment. Once they identify the key drivers of the business, they build the performance measurement system around those key elements. Whether called a scorecard, a performance measurement system, or just a set of metrics, the tool reflects what your business and organization strategy is all about. Figure 3.2 shows a beginning format for a balanced-scorecard tool.

Making the Scorecard Effective

To bring the balanced scorecard to life in your organization, incorporate the following eight actions:

1. *Establish high targets and stretch goals.* For example, aim for the 95th percentile on Customer satisfaction. Use it as a stimulus to excite people, and remember that small goals are not motivating. Find the balance between stretch and reasonableness.
2. *Keep it simple.* Have no more than three to four measures per objective area.

3. *Share measured information openly.* Move past the discomfort of having people see current numbers that may not be flattering. Place a wall-size board in the cafeteria with large departmental scorecards. Persevere through the period of initial confusion as to how departments connect to the organization's objectives, bringing

Figure 3.2—Balanced Scorecard

Organizational Goals				
High Satisfaction				
Objectives	**Measures**	**Target for Year**	**Current Performances**	**Initiatives**
KRA*: Customer satisfaction				
High Quality				
Objectives	**Measures**	**Target for Year**	**Current Performances**	**Initiatives**
KRA: Quality				
Low Cost				
Objectives	**Measures**	**Target for Year**	**Current Performances**	**Initiatives**
KRAs: Productivity, economics				
Best People				
Objectives	**Measures**	**Target for Year**	**Current Performances**	**Initiatives**
KRAs: People growth, organization climate, innovation				

*KRA = Key result area

that piece on-stream later if necessary.

4. *Make goal labels user friendly.* Use common language and state goals in challenging terms.

5. *Connect goals to people.* For example, put labels for the four targets on a coffee mug, call the mug your "strategic plan," and teach the plan to the organization.

6. *Use best-people measures universally.* Measure the following by department and organization totals:
   - Training hours per Associate
   - Job satisfaction and morale
   - Implementation of Associates' ideas

7. *Drive change with the scorecard.* When managers report they cannot get their numbers due to barriers, remove the barriers.

8. *Tie goal achievement to compensation, rewards, and recognition.* Performance data serve to identify both stars and laggards.

Treat tough targets and their measures as an evolving system. As people work under a goal-measured system, they will see areas to improve and refine. There is no perfect implementation moment—so get started now.

QUESTIONS FOR THE LEADER

1. How satisfied are you with how your organization meets its objectives? Would the high-performance hospital model more adequately meet your needs?

2. Do Associates have a system to easily interact with management and to change work systems? Do you have measures that show this is happening in sufficient volume?

3. Are you prepared to receive pushback for setting higher standards?

4. Are your organization's values tied to job descriptions so that people see the connection between what they do and organizational results?

5. Are rewards and recognition for goal achievement adequate?

REFERENCES

Collins, J. 2001. *Good to Great: Why Some Companies Make the Leap...and Others Don't.* New York: HarperCollins.

Conference Board. 2005. "U.S. Job Satisfaction Keeps Falling, the Conference Board Reports Today." Press release. [Online article; retrieved 6/1/07.] http://www.conference-board.org/utilities/pressDetail.cfm?press_ID=2582.

Kaplan, R., and D. Norton. 1996. *The Balanced Scorecard: Translating Strategy into Action.* Boston: Harvard Business School Press.

Nohria, N., W. Joyce, and B. Robertson. 2003. "What Really Works." *Harvard Business Review* 81 (7): 42–52. [Online article; retrieved 6/1/06.] http://www.willer.ca/steve/articles/what-really-works/.

Reagan, R. 1981. First inaugural address. [Online information; retrieved 6/28/07.] http://www.reaganfoundation.org/reagan/speeches/first.asp.

Rigby, D., and B. Bilodeau. 2007. *Management Tools and Trends 2007.* Boston: Bain & Company. [Online information; retrieved 6/28/07.] http://www.bain.com/bainweb/PDFs/cms/Public/Management%20Tools%202007%20BB.pdf.

CHAPTER 4

The Effectiveness Prescription

"Don't get buried in the thick of thin things."

—Stephen Covey

You can learn the behaviors of managerial effectiveness and can improve team and organization performance. Defining the job of management becomes a key ingredient to moving forward.

WINNERS AND LOSERS IN MANAGEMENT

GSM only happens with gold standard managers. Key to attaining GSM performance is the reassignment of managers who are currently ineffective in their tasks. They may be wonderful people, but their performance in management is marginal. Effectiveness is the primary requirement in management work, because only effectiveness makes it possible to get things ▶

done through other people. There is a range of managerial performance, with some effective managers at the high end of the distribution, and some marginal or failed managers at the bottom end of the distribution. Does your organization have people in management who should be removed or who need substantial retreading? What percent would you estimate? Unless that number is very small, you are looking at the primary reason why the organization struggles.

Risks of Ineffectiveness

Simply stated, no organization can afford any weak managers. Some organizations, like General Electric, conduct annual systematic culling, removing the 10 percent of managers with the weakest performance. The practice is controversial to some, but there is no question that it removes the weakest of the weak.

Left untended, the problem of subpar managerial performance can represent millions of dollars in liability, deaths of patients, and even the death of the organization. Managers are ineffective because of a number of known causes: selection error, lack of training and development, poor bosses, lack of

consequences, and apathy toward the problem.

WHAT MAKES A MANAGER EFFECTIVE?

The good news is that we know the success profile of effective managers. We know where they come from and how to assist their development. To a large degree, you can imitate and copy that profile, and you can even require it of your management team.

What Predicts Effective Managers?

What is predictive in the histories of people who win in management (Judge et al. 1995)? What is related to their ability to get results? The answers to these questions relate to childhood.

The first major indicator is that effective managers typically had childhoods where they had to work, often because of lower socio-economic circumstances. They had jobs in adolescence, if not caused by financial need then required by smart parents. They learned to work earlier than many of their peers. As adults, they do not shrink from hard work.

A second element of their childhood may include being first in the birth order, where expectations were higher than for later siblings or where they were put in charge of younger children (and reported to the CEO known as Mom or Dad) (Crittenden 2004). Variations on this theme include being the firstborn child of their gender in the family, or first in a much later generation of children.

The third element is that successful managers are smart; they always have above average IQ scores, but they are not necessarily brilliant or at genius level (Menkes 2005). Being an effective manager requires mental horsepower of a particular kind. People described as having "common sense" or "street smarts" seem to do well in management. Effective managers characteristically have a practical or applied approach to problems rather than an academic approach. No organization can give common sense to people—it can only find people with common sense through careful selection.

A final element found in the childhood experience of effective managers is that they often had experience in scouts, athletics, or another organized youth program that follows the basic model of *learning* a task, *doing* the task, and *being rewarded* for task mastery.

This cycle teaches people the joy of achievement. Achievement teaches self-confidence, a feeling that one can do anything that he is willing to learn and practice.

What Are the Secrets of Success?

SECRET 1. Regardless of how a person's past life was structured, in the present there is one element that predicts success more than any other—the desire to win. Personality psychologists tell us that the need for achievement acts as a driving force, pushing the individual toward the goal lines that matter to them (Raven 2001). We see this desire to achieve in persons with disabilities, athletes, firefighters, or anyone who rises above adversity to meet a challenge. In less dramatic form, GSM leaders identify the drive in their staff and create circumstances where that drive can be mobilized.

Some people will persist to the goal, while others simply fold. Winning leaders know that the will to win is not something you can give someone. You must find people who are wired that way. Thus, there is a substantial cottage industry attempting to assess motivation and personality. Selection testing makes sense and is worth the cost. Barring psychological assessment, look for a clear track record of past achievement in multiple aspects of living, because that pattern is likely to carry over into their management job.

SECRET 2. The second secret of effective managers is that they do the management job in different ways from their ineffective counterparts. Effective managers approach the arenas of time, work, people, priorities, and decisions differently. Their approaches achieve better results.

The skills used in their approaches are learned either by trial and error or under the tutelage of an effective manager. The good news is that you can teach these techniques, and anyone can learn to do them. It is in this arena that an organization can tool up its leadership team and expect greater results improvement.

Effective techniques are simple, contrarian, and disciplined:

- *Simple:* The techniques are not difficult to learn.
- *Contrarian:* While commonsensible, the techniques are often not readily apparent and are outside the proverbial box.

They make sense, but often are against conventional wisdom.
- *Disciplined:* Their power lies in their consistent application.

What Is Not Predictive of Managerial Success

Effective managers are not predictive by age, gender, ethnicity, or religion. These demographic details matter little. Harder to understand is that neither education nor grade point average is predictive of success. Having a college degree, including MBA or MHA credentials, may have value, but it does not make a manager effective (O'Reilly 1994). A great deal of reexamination is under way in academia to explain why formal education in management does not seem to directly correlate to organization performance (Pfeffer and Fong 2002). Management requires work and edge more than academics. As Mark Twain put it, "Never let your schooling interfere with your education." Effective managers avoid that trap.

Also, one's ability to get results is not directly related to personality (Boudreau, Boswell, and Judge 2001). While it is more enjoyable to work with a nice manager than a nasty one, the goal is getting results. It may be uncomfortable to consider,

> **Rx FOR SUCESS**
>
> Results = Achievement drive + Effectiveness practices

but tough bosses like General Patton could get results when others could not. This is not an argument against being good with people or skilled in relationships, it is simply an observation that personality alone is not predictive of results.

12 KEY HABITS FOR RESULTS

The most basic realization coming from the studies of managerial effectiveness is that success results from doing fewer things, but doing them extremely well (Boyatzis 1982). Effective managers and their teams work more selectively. They identify the vital few tasks associated with key results and focus on those. The organization can do without a lot of stuff; what it cannot do without is work that contributes to key business results.

The Pareto Principle notes that 80 percent of results come from only 20 percent of the items on the manager's desk. The trap lies in the 80 percent of items known as the "trivial many"—most of the paper in your in-basket and documentation related to meetings that contribute virtually nothing to end results. Effective managers sift out the elements that matter (Bruch et al. 2006).

Effective managers are not clones. They are not identical in how they go about their work, but they do have similar behaviors (Kotter 1999). Effective managers use 12 key habits to keep on track toward results:

Work Approach

1. *Be ruthless with time.* Effective managers do not wish for more time; they know they already have all the time there is. They use their time on tasks that matter and turn down requests that devote time to marginal activity, like most meetings. They close their doors to drop-in visitors and adjust their time to spend 5 percent to 10 percent more time on key results area (KRA) work.

2. *Stick to priorities.* Setting priorities is easy. The trick is to stay with those priorities and protect them from all the things that would be nice to do but that drag away from things that matter most.

3. *Gate work.* Effective managers do not try to win favors by agreeing to do everything that people ask of them. They say no to useless work. They gate into their department tasks that contribute to key results and fend off tasks that do not. For nonresults work

that must be done, such as regulatory requirements, do them quickly or delegate them.

Business Focus

4. *Act with urgency.* Move, move, move. A towering in-basket is not a sign of importance. Effective managers need a sense of urgency. Slow-as-molasses cultures often reveal ineffective management.

5. *Get to yes.* Effective managers are dealmakers. They create workable compromises. If they cannot get everything they want, they focus on what is possible now. They must sell their ideas to those in power.

6. *Wear a CEO mantle.* Successful managers see themselves as acting on behalf of their boss's boss. "If she were here, I think this is what she would do." They speak as though they own the place and thereby push the work forward.

Team Impacts

7. *Grow people.* Effective managers hire people smarter and more talented than themselves. They turn people loose to solve problems. The return on investment from that effort is a jump in results.

8. *Create synergy/energy.* No matter how much intelligence and drive the effective manager represents, he understands that relationships with staff and colleagues multiply that power. Effective managers find ways to work with others that increase mutual gain.

9. *Release ideation.* Each person on payroll has a brain. Effective managers elicit and solicit the thinking of everyone around them using this creative juice to generate energy. This may be the most critical requirement for organizational success. The effective manager knows that real power lies in finding ways to say yes to the creative thinking in others.

Inner Person

10. *Manage self.* Effective managers practice self-management and discipline. They control anger, show up on time, meet deadlines, and refrain from telling offensive stories or acting sexist. They practice good health habits and are people of character and ethic. They know that the first person they have to manage is themselves.

11. *Be proactive.* Effective people are fire preventers, not fire responders. Effective managers focus on what can be done rather than on the barriers that exist.

12. *Be a warrior with a mission.* Effective leaders do not play at their profession. They see purpose in their life and possess the spirit of the warrior and a sense of mission. Their passion for what they do is infectious; it spreads to those around them. There is joy in their labor.

PRESCRIPTIONS FOR EFFECTIVENESS

GSM requires the use of effective management techniques. The following is a condensed list of GSM practices that produce results. Put a check mark by those practices you or your team could improve upon and begin a development plan:

Contribution Focus
❒ Focus personal and subordinates' efforts on significant areas of contribution and away from trivia and meaningless work
❒ Survey Customers/users of products/services, determine their reactions to the unit's output, and modify to suit Customer needs
❒ Evaluate projects for their business value, meaningfulness, and economic justification; do not do work because it is there
❒ Push for productivity improvements through better technology, work systems, Associate training, and performance measurement
❒ Improve the organization climate through team building, fair Associate treatment, socialization, and emphasis on quality of work life
❒ Maintain GSM standards of performance and an orientation to excellence as prime job requirements

Time Management
❒ Regularly invest at least one hour a day working on your most important project—a KRA hour—where phone calls and other interruptions are blocked
❒ Invest 5 percent to 10 percent of your time thinking through what needs to be done and what needs to be stopped
❒ Focus on accomplishing the more important issues, not on simply reacting to the urgent issues (The important is seldom urgent.)

- Look for recurrent crises to find system errors and correct them through better forms design, training, more complete delegation, or other appropriate measures to prevent problem recurrence
- Enforce discipline in meeting management (e.g., starting on time, using agendas, having a chairperson), or voice your opinion that meeting management is needed
- Regularly say no to requests from subordinates, peers, and bosses to do work that will not contribute significantly to results

Priorities for the Future
- Concentrate on what is needed to be effective now and in the future rather than on problems that come from systems designed to serve the past
- Remain flexible to changing realities, but also successfully protect priorities by refusing to do the unnecessary things people want you to do
- Regularly recommend that programs, policies, or project clutter be eliminated or reduced to keep the unit trim
- Keep people on projects where they will have a maximum impact upon significant results and effectiveness
- Establish priorities with courage, identifying what is significant versus what is easy to do
- Keep people's priorities limited to two or three objectives in the current period; do not continuously throw more at them

Build on Strengths
- Build on the strengths of Associates by focusing on what they can do instead of worrying about what they cannot do
- Put people in jobs that require them to stretch and grow rather than remain static
- Delegate consistently to subordinates, giving them full authority and freedom to take action to develop them and free yourself for more important tasks
- Expect people to get the right things done, not simply be busy
- Ruthlessly challenge any policy, procedure, or other artificial limitation that prevents staff from achieving their fullest potential
- Reserve the toughest tasks for yourself, and accomplish at least one significant item daily

Managerial Communications
- Let subordinates and others know how you feel as a person as well as a boss so you are viewed as authentic

□ Provide systematic reinforcement and recognition each day to signal to others how they are doing

□ Quickly provide reprimanding, yet face-saving, correction when it is needed so Associates are warned of performance deviation

□ Ask for recommendations from staff, but do not provide answers to problems for them

□ Avoid giving overlapping assignments to Associates to prevent duplication of effort and useless competition

□ Communicate with clarity, directness, timeliness, relevance, brevity, and action

Managing Results

□ Mutually establish the work agenda with your boss, blending organization objectives with your own

□ Show sensitivity to individual needs and goals, blending staff work needs with organizational goals

□ Give assignments completely: set project priorities; specify what is to be done; identify standards that will measure acceptable performance; set progress review and completion dates; spell out levels of authority; and ask for staff commitment

□ Keep staff constantly up to date with new information on changing problems, needs, and objectives

□ Systematically identify and eliminate roadblocks that prevent staff from performing, and provide political as well as logistical support

□ Share periodic performance appraisal information with Associates so they know how they are doing against project checkpoints and how you react to their work

Action Decision Making

□ Make decisions logically and rationally by gathering as much data as budget and time will allow, and only then apply the test of your judgment or gut instinct in reaching a conclusion

□ Draw on the experience and wisdom of others by listening to and involving those who are closest to the problem

□ Ask for multiple problem solution alternatives, or spark a debate among advisers to avoid the error of groupthink

□ Delegate everything that people reporting to you can do, should do, or could be trained to do, refusing to make decisions they could make

❑ Encourage staff to be success-seekers and risk-takers rather than failure-avoiders and check-firsters

❑ Move rapidly in making decisions to keep action pacing alive, and move slowly only on those few decisions that are hard to reverse

Personal Managerial Development

❑ Invest in good personal health practices: have annual physicals; watch eating, smoking, and drinking habits; and follow an adequate exercise program

❑ Pursue ongoing professional development through reading, formal classroom work, on-the-job learning, and understudying mentors

❑ Establish a role as a "crucial subordinate," one truly needed by at least two in-house sponsors who can further your project and career interests

❑ Deal comfortably with authority figures, and react to your boss's needs with understanding

❑ Build bridges rather than drive wedges between people, handling conflict situations assertively rather than passively or aggressively

❑ Analyze causes of project or personal failure to face the facts, determine future actions, and bounce back with resiliency

Using this list as an inventory instrument, hospital managers typically score highest on Managerial Communications and Build on Strengths, categories that suggest they are good in people relationships. Weakest scores are usually in the categories of Time Management, and Priorities for the Future. The combined profile suggests hospital managers are generally nice people, but lagging in work outputs and providing mediocre results.

For most managers, the GSM cure is management education in effectiveness techniques, installation of an organization-wide management system that supports those practices, and performance evaluation system that removes those who choose not to follow the path toward results.

QUESTIONS FOR THE LEADER

1. Are you and your management team practicing management in a way that aligns with the effectiveness profile?

2. Does your organization spell out how managers should do their job and provide a way to remove those who are unable to do that job effectively?

REFERENCES

Boudreau, J. W., W. R. Boswell, and T. A. Judge. 2001. "Effects of Personality on Executive Career Success in the United States and Europe." *Journal of Vocational Behavior* 58 (1): 53–81.

Boyatzis, R. E. 1982. *The Competent Manager: A Model for Effective Performance*. New York: Wiley.

Bruch, H., S. Ghosal, W. Oncken, Jr., D. L. Wass, S. R. Covey, and R. S. Kaplan. 2006. *Habits of Highly Effective Managers*, 2nd ed. *Harvard Business Review* OnPoint Collection. Boston: Harvard Business School Publishing.

Crittenden, A. 2004. *If You've Raised Kids, You Can Manage Anything: Leadership Begins at Home*. New York: Gotham.

Judge, T., D. M. Cable, J. W. Boudreau, and R. D. Bretz, Jr. 1995. "An Empirical Investigation of the Predictors of Executive Career Success." *Personnel Psychology* 48 (3): 485–519.

Kotter, J. P. 1999. "What Effective General Managers Really Do." *Harvard Business Review* 77 (2): 145-156.

Menkes, J. "Hiring for Smarts." 2005. *Harvard Business Review* (83) 11: 100–109.

O'Reilly, B. 1994. "Reengineering the MBA." *Fortune*, January 24.

Pfeffer, J., and C. T. Fong. 2002. "The End of Business Schools? Less Success Than Meets the Eye." *Academy of Management Learning and Education* 1 (1): 78–95. [Online article; retrieved 6/1/07.] http://www.gmac.com/NR/rdonlyres/12D258C6-F3B1-4AFF-A3B5-1158B8F2E820/0/Pfefferarticle.pdf.

Raven, J. 2001. "The McClelland/McBer Competency Models." In *Competence in the Learning Society*, edited by J. Raven and J. Stephenson. New York: Peter Lang.

CHAPTER 5

A System for Winning

"It's all very well in practice, but it will never work in theory."

—French management saying

Once you figure out how to do something well, the key is to document it, teach it to users, and require adherence. The choices in management are simple—either manage with a system that handles some of the workload for you, or try to manage the uncontrolled situation that inevitably results when management has no systematic approach to getting work done.

PLAYING TO WIN

Effective organizations define what works for them and insist that all management follow this approach. This is the core of systems thinking, and nowhere is it more required than in defining ▶

how managers manage. If you want your team to succeed, you need to clearly define their objectives and tasks. For example, it is clear that a key to success at Marriott Corporation is their management approach (Marriott and Zackheim 1997):

> At the most basic level, systems help bring order to the natural messiness of human enterprise. Give 100 people the same task—without providing ground rules—and you'll end up with at least a dozen, if not 100, different ways of doing it. Try that same experiment with a few thousand people, and you end up with chaos.... I'm always a little surprised when I come across companies that aren't as devoted to [systems] as we are. I often see wasted opportunities to improve performance, simply because no one seems to be focusing on developing, much less implementing and maintaining, systems and standards.

That is GSM thinking! Whether described in Sam Walton's book, *Made in America*, Southwest Airline's *Nuts!*, or Jack Welch's *Winning*, successful executives articulate their approaches to management and require their teams to follow them. Successful hospital leaders do the same.

A Management System Removes Variance

Too much management variance inevitably creates conflict and downtime that is costly and risky. Similar to having a financial system, an information management system, or a patient care system, having a management system makes it easier to get things done. Said another way, without a management system, chances of success are small. Common terminology, tools, procedures, and philosophies remove detrimental management variance and confusion and free the team for productive contribution.

MANSYS: AN EXAMPLE MANAGEMENT SYSTEM

Let us examine one type of management system called MANSYS. MANSYS is an example of GSM tools, time lines, and processes that all managers would use in an organization. Many of the tools can be tailored to fit your organization, and users may want to add other tools. The point is that all management issues and processes are addressed in a management practices manual, and all managers are expected to apply these standardized tools. MANSYS brings new managers quickly up to speed on how pieces of management work are done at your organization, and it brings the most experienced manager into a framework that puts her on the same wavelength as the rest of the team.

MANSYS content is derived from the work habits and techniques used by effective managers—those producing more results than their ineffective counterparts. As a systematic approach, MANSYS can be used as a first draft for developing your in-house managing system. What every organization needs is a system that spells out (1) how to be effective, (2) where management's focus should be, (3) the centrality of good people management, (4) the structured elements that control work results, and (5) how to deal with change. MANSYS is about how to do the management job and "how we do it around here." MANSYS involves five key concepts: being effective, staying focused, leading people, managing work, and driving change. At the website for Gold Standard Management, you can access MANSYS manual, forms, and instructions (goldstandard management.org/ACHE/MANSYS. html).

CHECKLIST FOR MANAGEMENT SYSTEM IMPLEMENTATION

To effectively implement your own in-house management system, follow these five easy steps:

1. Create a project team to review elements of a proposed management system that all managers would use. Start with existing management systems that others have written, like MANSYS, and edit from there. Make recommendations for the topical headings and proposed tools for executive review.
2. Decide which chapters/concepts will be core requirements for all managers and which are optional. Core practices must include creating quarterly or monthly work plans (management by objectives) and meeting management rules.
3. Prune out existing forms, procedures, and practices that are ineffective so they do not

become part of the new management system.

4. Prepare a document called "The President's Guide to Management Success." Some executives simply create a list of expected managerial dos and don'ts. Some executives insert several pages of their philosophy—this is essential because it defines the new management culture.

5. Schedule management training to introduce the new management tools and expectations and also articulate those management processes that have been deleted.

QUESTIONS FOR THE LEADER

1. Will a standardized system of management tools and process based upon best practices aid our management team?

2. Who will lead the initiative to adopt GSM processes and tools? How quickly can this be undertaken?

REFERENCES

Freidberg, K. L., and J. A.Freidberg. 1996. *Nuts!: Southwest Airline's Crazy Recipe for Business and Personal Success*. New York: Broadway.

Marriott, J. W., and A. Zackheim. 1997. *Spirit to Serve: Marriott's Way*. New York: Harper Collins.

Walton, S., and J. Huey. 1992. *Sam Walton: Made in America*. New York: Bantam.

Welch, J., and S. Welch. 2005. *Winning*. New York: HarperCollins.

CHAPTER 6

The Gold Standard Management Audit

"The quality of a leader is reflected in the standards they set for themselves.

—Ray Kroc, McDonald's Founder

I f you want to win, do what winners do. Following every football game, coaches make teams look at game films to spot areas for improvement. After every military engagement, U.S. Army units conduct an after-action review. When was the last time your management team took a hard look at itself to find a better way forward?

WHAT NEEDS REVIEW?

Studies show that high-performance organizations spend considerable time defining how they manage, and as a consequence have improved business results in subsequent periods (de Waal 2005). To stay on top of things, effective leaders conduct quarterly reviews of how they are ▶

managing. This is the action-oriented, and sometimes uncomfortable, work of deciding who and what needs to change. This leads to shedding wasted performance and projects, and improves the rate at which the organization adapts.

AUDITING PERFORMANCE RESULTS

A basic doctrine of effective management is that how results are obtained is relatively unimportant as long as there are no legal or values violations. If downstream results are not being adequately produced, then upstream processes need to change. Use the following suggested GSM minimum performance standards to audit your organization's current performance and to determine what additional activity needs to be added to your organization to operate at GSM levels.

While the GSM audit incorporates measures of both end results and the management processes that produced them, there is more focus on outcomes than on the upstream processes that produce them. Following are some of the performance outcomes that indicate an organization is on track. Add to the list to reflect additional special needs of your situation. Is your organization hitting as many of these outcomes as it needs to?

High Customer Satisfaction:
- Organization Customer ratings are at the 95th percentile or greater compared to a norm group (use a large database to ensure hard comparisons).

High Quality—satisfied by any one of the following:
- The organization ranks in the 90th percentile on HCIA-Mercer or other tough quality indicators.
- The organization appears on the *Solucient* Top 100 Hospitals list.
- The Leapfrog Group's three prime indicators of computerized order entry, hospitalists, and volume of surgeries requirement are met.[1]

Low Cost—satisfied by any of the following:
- Prices have been frozen to market for two to three years in a row.
- The organization ranks in the 90th percentile on HCIA-Mercer cost indicators.

Best People—all of the following must be met:
- All Associates spend 40 hours per year on training. All forms of training and orientation are included.

- Overall staff morale scores at the 90th percentile for the core questions: "My overall rating of my job" and "I would recommend a good friend to work here."
- Ideation implementation equals or exceeds three ideas per person during each calendar year.

Performance outcomes like these suggest that while operational imperfections may remain, it is likely that many current management processes are working. However, no leader can ever be sure of that. Many of the best leaders worry to the point of paranoia that today's successes may be making the organization too comfortable and that seeds of tomorrow's problems may already be growing.

EXAMINING UPSTREAM MANAGEMENT PROCESSES

If results are unsatisfactory, the fix is changing how you manage. The decision rule would look like this:

If results are bad, the problem stems from poor management processes.

If results are good, something may still be wrong with management's approach.

The following is a list of GSM practices that contribute to organizational success. Use this checklist to determine whether something is missing in your organization's management practices:

Balanced Scorecard
- Balanced scorecards are posted prominently in public and department areas.
- Goals are at audacious levels similar to those required for results.
- Measures used are both valid and have credible databases.
- Dates for accomplishment are set for 12 to 24 months, not long time periods.
- Substantial annual tactical work plans are rolled out under a commando change group, charged with implementation. Commandos are given substantial authority to make change aggressively—a plum assignment!

Leader Selection
- Leaders are selected less for technical skills and more for interpersonal skills and achievement of results.

- Leaders are selected for edge, execution, energy, and energizing capabilities, and they are in line with the predictive profile elements found in effective performers (see Chapter 4).
- Leaders are selected using a formal and intensive selection process.

Leadership Education and Evaluation
- The management team completes a substantial amount of managerial education annually on topics considered fundamental and contemporary to the field.
- Instructors must be competent, evaluated annually, and replaced as necessary.
- Managers are evaluated by staff, peers, and executives in some form of 360-degree process.

Management System
- A comprehensive house-wide management system details organizational values, philosophy, and management operating practices beyond those normally found in personnel and accounting manuals.

Time Management
- Ninety percent of meetings are controlled with a prioritized agenda and start and stop times, and they are paced and evaluated for results.
- Nonproductive meetings or committees follow a sundown rule—too few results put the group out of existence.
- Seventy-five percent of middle management meetings with executives are used for upward communication on operating problems and needs. Most executive announcements are relegated to print or email.
- All managers use KRA hours to focus on priority problems or needs at least four days per week.
- Reduction of paperwork, processes, and other trivial tasks is aggressively pursued.

Work Planning and Organization
- Projects considered essential to business mission are identified in each area in sufficient quantity to "move the numbers."
- The management team uses some form of management by objectives in which a written list of KRA tasks is prioritized, agreed upon, and followed up by involved executives. This procedure is repeated on a monthly or quarterly basis. An annual work list does not qualify.
- Tasks noncontributory to key results are minimized, delegated

only if there is a positive development consequence to the person asked to do them, or are automated.

Tools and Systems

- Productivity is enhanced by adequate investment in tools, technology, and systems.
- Flowcharting, travel time calculations, work simplification, and process improvement efforts are substantially underway.
- Standards are set; second-rate vendors, equipment, and supplies are not used.
- Variance in performance and cost are removed by standardizing how things are done clinically and managerially.

People Resources

- Selection of staff follows the rule of best person, and they are selected by multiple raters in multiple interviews. Vacancies are left open if qualified candidates are not available.
- Problem people who cannot be developed are quickly removed.
- Substantial recognition and reward are routinely provided to all staff.
- Small-group process and participation are widespread.

- "Every employee, a manager" is practiced, and empowerment is high.
- "Open book" management is practiced.

The aforementioned practices above are not all that could be considered. Users at the outset are best served with a short list of processes and outcomes as presented here. Invariably, successful organizations add and refine both process and results criteria as they continue to progress. The need is to be centered on results and the processes that drive them. Then, check on how the overall revitalization effort is coming together. It establishes focus in the midst of myopia.

REWARD RESULTS TO DRIVE CHANGE

By rewarding departments that carry out GSM practices, the effect will be to reinforce the new management culture. Internally, executives could give the following GSM awards:

- *Management Process Achievement Award.* This four-star award is recognition for instituting a substantial body of management best practices that are expected to yield results within the year. Points would be awarded for the degree to which correct management procedures are followed, problem issues removed, etc. A process achievement award is only an interim marker on the road to GSM performance.

- *Results Achievement Award.* This is a five-star award. Results are at acceptable GSM levels for each of the four measured outcomes of quality, cost, Customer, and people. Points are awarded solely for results, not effort.

QUESTIONS FOR THE LEADER

1. Who should be assigned the task of conducting your GSM audit?

2. What sequence of consequences will be employed with managers who are not following GSM practices?

3. How will your leadership team drive an award process to aid motivation toward GSM performance outcomes?

NOTE

1. Leapfrog Group. 2007. "What Does Leapfrog Ask Hospitals?" [Online information; retrieved 6/1/07.] http://www.leapfroggroup.org/for_consumers/hospitals_asked_what.

REFERENCE

de Waal, A. A. 2005. *The Characteristics of a High Performance Organization.* Paper presented at the British Academy of Management Conference, Oxford, UK, Sept. 13–15. [Online paper; retrieved 1/7/07.] http://www.andredewaal.nl/pdf/Bam2005.pdf.

ENERGY

CHAPTER 7

Building Managerial Muscle

"Before you are a leader, success is all about growing yourself. When you become a leader, success is all about growing others."

—Jack Welch, former CEO of GE

Newton's first law observes that a body at rest stays at rest unless acted upon by an outside force. The organizational landscape is littered with failed change efforts, and today's ballyhooed project is likely to be tomorrow's failed program of the month. Inertia is a common evil in organizational management. The change leader understands that force, and energy must be applied if things are to change.

Energy that is applied in a sustained, sensible, directed manner begins to move the organization. Movement is slow at first, and then it gathers speed until a forward momentum is achieved. When you break the forces of inertia, the biggest part of the problem is behind you because then there is a flywheel of force that only needs to be nurtured. ▸

WHY DEVELOP LEADERS?

It is important to understand why managers produce inadequate results in spite of working hard. Figure 7.1 shows the performance scores of a typical hospital management team on two key dimensions: their

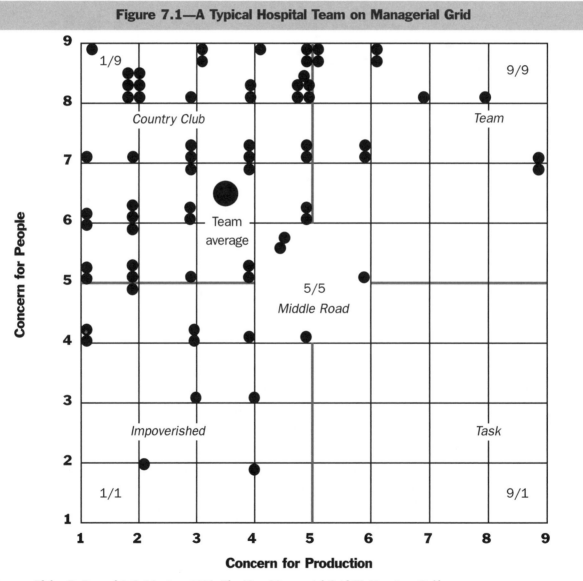

Figure 7.1—A Typical Hospital Team on Managerial Grid

Source: Blake, R. R., and J. S. Mouton. 1985. *The New Managerial Grid III*. Houston: Gulf.

orientation toward *people* (consideration) and *production* (structure). The model is known as the managerial grid (Blake and Mouton 1985), a widely used organization diagnostic. The profile shown is typical of hospital management teams—a picture endemic to the industry. Think of this graph as a beginning picture of where your organization may be currently. Your organization might be in any one of the quadrants shown in Figure 7.1:

- *Country-club organizations* result when managers have a high concern for people and a low concern for production. This makes for a comfortable and friendly organization, but work output and quality suffers. Such organizations are facing economic uncertainty.
- *Task organizations* represents the opposite of a country-club organization. Here, managers are so focused on getting the work out that relationships suffer and tend to break down into hostility and conflict. In extreme cases, labor-law violations and union conflict can ensue.
- *Impoverished organizations* have so little of both factors that this

quadrant often represents poor performance and future failure.
- *Team organizations*, like a championship team, have both camaraderie and rapid-flow performance. The interactions are fluid, and both staff and organizational interests are well served. This is the quadrant of best-in-industry high performance.
- *Middle-road organizations* have achieved a balance that enables them to function, but they are never going to achieve high performance. They do enough positive things for people and get enough work done that they are able to muddle through. Most organizations fall in this category.

Successful organizations exist only in the upper right quadrant (team organization). All others are in various states of decay and have questionable futures. The task of the leader is to move the management team to a performance level representing both a high concern for people (the consideration and connection they need) and a high concern for production (the structure required to get work done).

The management team in Figure 7.1 is in the counrty-club quadrant and is struggling with performance results. Two problems are illustrated. First, this team's average score is too low on production—organizational outputs of quantity and quality are suffering. The second problem hospital management teams typically experience is an extreme variance among the opinions of leaders. The variance in leadership opinion literally pulls the organization apart. Open feuding may not be present, but a lack of cohesion exists, and common views about how to manage are missing. Of special note are the following:

- In the example, the team's primary need is for increased orientation toward production, sometimes referred to as structure. It is reasonable to conclude that management members need time management skills, work systems improvement, problem-Associate management skills, and an accountability framework.
- Some individual scores are so low on both dimensions as to point toward a selection error in placing these people into management. While scores can be improved somewhat, the distance from a score of one on production to an acceptable score of five represents two standard deviations. This

great a variation suggests that the manager is unlikely to become effective even with heavy management education.

Management development is done to build the business. In this typical hospital picture, the variance in management approaches must be narrowed to result in greater alignment and increased functionality and performance. Failing that, the organization is doomed to mediocrity.

Improving the Management Mix

Following are six strategies to align your managers:

1. *Hire selectively.* Select leaders with both a strong approach to concern for people and concern for production.
2. *Fire quickly.* Remove managers who are weak on these two dimensions. A caveat: While ideal candidates are in short supply, it is more effective to work short handed until proper candidates can be found.
3. *Develop managers.* A requirement is that educational effort must be substantial and

repeated annually—it is not a one-shot, one-day event. A caveat: Training can fill in knowledge deficiencies and change attitudes, but experience shows the gain from training will not exceed 10 percent. Do not expect to remake people. 4. *Set expectations.* Use the Leader's Credo (Appendix A) to unify expectations among all managers. Have all managers sign a copy for their employment files and post it in every management meeting.

5. *Provide feedback.* Use Customer satisfaction, Associate satisfaction, and peer ratings feedback on areas of strength and developmental need. Feedback and targeted corrective action can change behavior.

6. *Reward system.* Tie consequences to managerial behaviors and results. Make bonuses or profit sharing a bigger part of the compensation pay plan. Set annual performance and educational requirements for recertification of membership in the "President's Management Academy" (a label that you can use to convey attainment as a professional within the organization).

IMPLEMENTING A COMMANDO COLLEGE

Goals of management development are clear: to build skill sets among managers that support high outputs and to unify the philosophy, priorities, and practices among the leadership team.

How much training do managers need? As a general statement, expenditures of time and money are loosely correlated with organizational performance: the more you spend, the more you get. Based on benchmarks from successful organizations and research into the amount of time required to impart core skills, a working number is 40 to 60 hours of classroom training in the first year and approximately 40 hours annually thereafter (Brown et al. 1998). Additional hours out of class are required for homework and assignments.

The following is a suggested course outline and sequence that is a workable platform for management development. Consider it a point of departure and revise as required. The course is based on 12 classroom days, arranged as six two-day sessions spread throughout one year. Assignments related to organization needs are completed between sessions.

As an example, when problem-Associate management is discussed as a classroom topic, the assignment is to create an action plan on each problem person so that the problem does not linger in the organization. In the following course sequence, place a checkmark next to topics you think would benefit your organization.

Session 1: Profiles in Excellence

Outcomes: Unify organizational mission and individual commitment to team goals, improve time and meeting management practices, and standardize professional management practices.

☐ *Day 1—Creating a High-Performance Hospital:* Describe the high-performance organization that leaders have decided to create, mobilize commitment to change, and identify targets where the organization can change and improve.

☐ *Day 2—Uncommon Leadership and Effectiveness:* Identify behaviors, practices, and techniques that yield results; profile each manager's level of effectiveness; and create an action plan to manage work, time, people, and priorities.

Session 2: The Power of People

Outcomes: Develop a tactical plan for employing the best people; install new management practices, better selection methods, and quality-of-life elements; identify required leadership behaviors and turnover causes for action; and create action plans for rehabilitating nonperformers.

☐ *Day 1—Leadership for Growth and Contribution:* Learn to tap the sources of motivation in today's Associates, and get people with you through motivation management and achievement/reward systems.

☐ *Day 2—Transforming Problem People:* Not everyone belongs on a championship team. Get nonperformers out of the organization or help them return to high performance levels.

Session 3: The Privilege of Service

Outcomes: Install a tactical plan to improve Customer service in your organization, and work on managerial performance issues and accountability.

☐ *Day 1—The Customer Is King:* There is no business success without satisfied Customers. Implement a complete strategy for Customer service, and learn how to let the Customer teach you your business.

❏ *Day 2—Accountability in Management:* Check to see that things get done, are done right, and are done on time; redeploy resources to solve problems instead of asking for more staff and budget; and eliminate excuses for nonperformance.

Session 4: Risking for Greatness

Outcomes: Increase initiative taking, reduce managers' dependency on executives, remove change resistance factors, and track ideation.

❏ *Day 1—Managerial Muscle, Power, and Persuasion:* Be politic without being political, get ideas sold within the organization, and press for new approaches without being offensive.

❏ *Day 2—Creativity and Controlling Change:* Change and innovation are essential to any organization's future. Learn to deal with resistance to change, use resistant energy in positive ways, and redefine conflict and use it for accomplishment.

Session 5: Quality, Speed, and Results

Outcomes: Establish common continuous improvement approaches as precursors to organization-wide training efforts, put slow total quality management (TQM) projects on short timelines, establish a tactical plan to develop high quality, and reduce the number and size of liability lawsuits.

❏ *Day 1—Continuous Improvement:* Overcome barriers to solving problems, and learn to master continuous improvement techniques and systematically solve work problems.

❏ *Day 2—Saving Time, Money, and Effort:* Master problem-solving and solution-implementation techniques; and implement lasting solutions and real fixes with better data usage and hard tools, like decision matrices and cycle-time analysis.

Session 6: Unifying Team Performance

Outcomes: Install productivity gains that outpace operating costs, improve speed of idea implementation, and reduce operating costs.

❏ *Day 1—Maximizing Productivity and Innovation:* Improve organization efficiency and conserve scarce resources while improving quality by investing in solid return on investment (ROI) tools and training.

❏ *Day 2—Building a Winning Team:* Learn and create characteristics of effective teams.

INTENSIFY KNOWLEDGE MANAGEMENT

The day of the corporate university is here. It is not just an expansion of the training department, but a set of new approaches to get knowledge solutions applied to the organization's work through the organization's people. Connect the management of new ideas to the educational function and develop a "Center for Learning and Innovation."

The conversion to Internet-based learning and repositories of best and updated work processes for each professional group is at hand. Briefly, the organization's response has to be the addition of education, organizational development, and process improvement staff. The offset is the substantial gains in productivity that these disciplines bring by spreading knowledge to the entire organization. Managerial muscle stems from having better-prepared and more-suited leaders and from increasing attention given to worker capabilities in an applied science business.

QUESTIONS FOR THE LEADER

1. Where would you estimate your team scores on the managerial grid? Do you observe problems with structure, such as missed deadlines, late-starting meetings, poor follow-through, and policy nonenforcement?
2. How can your organization integrate education and increase innovation by all staff to boost organization performance?
3. If money being spent on outside consultants as an idea source were spent on internal training, might the ROI be greater?

REFERENCES

Blake, R.R, and J. S. Mouton. 1985. *The Managerial Grid III.* Houston: Gulf.

Brown, K. G., C. C. Durham, A. L. Kristoff, L. Kunder, J. D. Olian, and R. M. Pierce. 1998. "Designing Management Training and Development for Competitive Advantage: Lessons from the Best." *Human Resource Planning* 21 (1): 20–31.

CHAPTER 8

Acres of Diamonds

"When the solution is simple, God is answering."

—Albert Einstein

U sing the considerable brainpower of an organization's people has proven to be more than sufficient to master its challenges. In the new era of hospital management, leaders are cutting the umbilical cord of consultant dependency and using the greater knowledge and capabilities of their own team. This strategy will be core to the success of healthcare.

FINDING YOUR TREASURE

R. H. Conwell (1960) tells the story of an ancient farmer, Ali Hafed, who dreams of discovering a field of diamonds that will make him rich beyond measure and transform his life. Even though ▶

Ali has much to make him content, the dream makes him feel poor in comparison to the wealth that might be his. He becomes obsessed with the idea of owning a diamond mine. As a result, he sells his farm and leaves his family to wander in search of diamonds. He finds nothing and eventually dies alone in true poverty.

This sad story has a second part. The man who purchases Ali's farm finds a number of odd stones and rocks. They do not appear to be of value, but he finds that they are indeed diamonds. He has discovered what would become India's Golconda diamond mine, a source of much wealth and some of the world's largest diamonds.

The moral of the fable: "Had Ali Hafed remained at home and dug in his own cellar, or underneath his own wheat fields or in his own garden, instead of wretchedness, starvation, and death by suicide in a strange land, he would have had 'acres of diamonds'" (Conwell 1960, 10).

Mining Your Diamond Field

The fable raises the question, are there acres of diamonds around today's leaders that they fail to see? Is it possible that those resources are actually "in the house" but are unrecognized? Could they be found in your own backyard, if you would only dig for them?

Management often fails to understand their management opportunity. An organization's biggest failing can be that it has not realized that its people are its prime competitive advantage. While a common sentiment of those in healthcare is that people are valuable, recognizing them as an asset is not the same as realizing their value. It is like knowing you have diamonds in the backyard, but not knowing how to extract them, how to cut and polish them, or how to distribute the final product to Customers.

Idea mining is the process of finding ideas for change and improvement. This is part of the new drive to focus on intellectual capital and knowledge management:

The most important, and indeed the truly unique, contribution of management in the 20th century was the fifty-fold increase in the productivity of the manual worker in manufacturing. The most important contribution management needs to make in the 21st century is similarly to increase the productivity of knowledge work and the knowledge worker (Drucker 1999, 135).

RELEASING INTELLECTUAL CAPITAL

GSM requires an organized system to collect Associate ideas. This is not an ineffective suggestion program, but rather an organization-wide approach that requires implementation of Associates' ideas. The following approach to increased ideation among staff can yield millions of dollars, even in its first year of implementation:

1. Require a specific number of implemented ideas per Associate per year. Three implemented ideas per person is a performance measure that can be obtained routinely by many healthcare organizations. Track ideation by Associate and department to spot productivity problems.
2. Implement 95 percent of ideas submitted, at least in part. This gives managers the ability to turn down a few ideas and requires them to work with the team to find ways to make their ideas work.
3. Establish a no-fail philosophy—there are no bad ideas. Thank Associates for submitting an idea. If the organization cannot accept an idea in full or can only

partially implement it, then thank the Associate for the contribution and encourage him to submit more ideas. Accompany this with a host of recognitions and rewards for ideas.
4. Require new training. One hour of training in a four-step problem-solving process called "DO IT" is required of all staff:
   - Define the problem
   - Outline options for solution
   - Implementation plan created
   - Track results
   The four-step process provides all staff with the same tools and processes for problem solving.
5. Lay out the rules: Solutions must be no cost or low cost, must fit the hospital's declared values and business objectives, and must be practical. You should implement nearly all ideas fitting these requirements. Compensation and benefit recommendations are off limits and are reserved to executive discretion.
6. Submit ROI estimates with each recommendation. Ideas that require substantial investment have a good chance for approval if the ROI picture is positive in the first 12 months. Many ideas are impossible to measure in terms of ROI, and they are

installed simply for their obvious business value.

7. All stakeholders affected by the solution are engaged in the process. The department manager approves problem solutions within their department. Ideas affecting other departments or that are interdepartmental go to a small task force, where they are managed with the input of stakeholders.

8. Participation in the ideation process is a prerequisite to future promotions or pay increases. Coming up with ways to improve things is not a tack-on job assignment. It is now a core part of everyone's job. People are paid to think and change the system, not simply to run yesterday's solutions.

An idea that can be developed and implemented by a single person—a JDI (Just Do It)—is carried out by the submitter or appropriate staff, with management assistance as needed. For example, if the location of egg-crate mattress storage on the nursing unit is changed, one person makes the change. When more than one person or department needs to address an issue, it becomes a DIG (Do It

Group). For example, if the repackaging sterile instruments could result in substantial savings, more than one department may need to be involved.

Idea Payoff

The experience of organizations implementing a JDI/DIG process shows that the average idea has a tangible ROI of $2,500–$4,000 in the first year. Calculate the average ROI by dividing the tangible ROI realized by the total number of implemented JDIs/DIGs, including those that have tangible ROI and those without. Estimate ROI at the time the proposal was submitted, and your financial management department evaluates and approves the ROI estimate.

EXERCISE. To get an estimate of the value of untapped intellectual capital in your organization, multiply the organization's headcount by three to get the number of ideas that your organization could reasonably expect to implement in the first year—your ideation budget. Then multiply that number by an assumed average ROI of $3,000. For example, a hospital of 1,200 Associates at three ideas per person could implement 3,600 ideas. With a tangible return of $3,000 per idea, the hospital could net approximately $10.8 million.

In practice, improvements often continue to have value in future years, but to be conservative and for practical ease there has been no attempt to track that phenomenon. The business platform spirals upward for improved operations in subsequent periods when an organization makes thousands of improvements annually.

The Baloney of "Low-Hanging Fruit"

A former criticism of this approach from the old TQM movement was that Associate ideas were "low-hanging fruit," a put-down of bubble-up ideation. Most of the fruit on a tree is low hanging, and fruit does not taste any better based on where it hangs. Never make the mistake of harvesting only high-hanging fruit!

Experience teaches that the JDI/DIG approach is an ideal way to begin unleashing and managing intellectual capital. At the end of the first year of training and ideation experience, you can introduce additional high-powered quality management tools and approaches as a *supplement* to overall ideation management and to address more

complicated processes. Some of the organization's defects are major and some are minor; under GSM, all are intolerable. The effective manager looks for solutions to all of his problems, not just those few deemed important. It is the sum of change made that counts, not whether the chunks of it were large or small.

TURNING ON THE CHANGE MACHINE

A key to any organization's future has always been its ability to manage change quickly and well. The new realization is that it must create change massively, not simply react to it, for being a large organization or having a successful history provides no security against competitors or a churning environment. In the new era, the swift will eat the slow. Time-based competition has become one of the new rules for market-share success. What is the turnaround time for making things happen in your organization?

As the evolution of healthcare continues to unfold, we find ourselves hampered by old organizational management approaches. Leaders need to do increasingly more, and they struggle to make change in a resistant, even dysfunctional, organization model.

Management today has concluded that the concept of the manager as the sole problem solver and decider simply will not work. To solve the speed problem, the new generation of hospital leaders knows that they have to radically alter the organization's operating system. That massive task can only be accomplished by dividing the work among the entire staff—not just the doing work, but the *thinking* work. This results in substantially more work done in a unit of time. Effective leaders are abandoning the concept of super-performing managers, who move with lightning speed to solve all problems, and embracing the idea that all Associates should think like management—that they are indeed managing. Therefore, the challenge of who deals with problems shifts from what a small group of managers can do to what the team at large can do. As all of the minds work the problems, the process becomes simplified and robust.

James Lincoln (1951), the American management genius who founded Lincoln Electric in 1895, put it this way:

It becomes perfectly true to anyone who will think this thing through that there is no such thing as a management activity, Management and Men having different functions or being two different kinds of people. Why can't we think and why don't we think that all people are Management? Can you imagine any president of any factory or machine shop who can go down and manage a turret lathe as well the machinist can? Can you imagine any manager of any organization who can go down and manage a broom—let us get down to that— who can manage a broom as well as a sweeper can?...Obviously, all are Management.

SUMMING UP

In an applied-science business, to think of Associates as diamonds is apt, especially when looking at the sparkling facets of their thinking. However, diamonds need a proper setting—a culture that values each contributor and provides a system to implement the thinking of so many minds. There are indeed acres of diamonds in the untapped thinking and contributions of healthcare professionals. It has been there all along; it just needs to be mined.

The success of GSM in improving hospital performance has been dramatic and consistent. It has repeatedly shown that future excellence does not depend on past reputation or current situation. It does not matter how little you have in the way of financial resources. It is all about the people you have, how they are led, and whether leaders understand what they must do.

A LAST QUESTION FOR THE LEADER

1. Healthcare is at a point of being ready for a significant upgrade in how it manages. Are you ready to lead it?

REFERENCES

Conwell, R. H. 1960. *Acres of Diamonds*. New York: Jove.

Drucker, P. F. 1999. *Management Challenges for the 21st Century*. New York: HarperCollins.

Lincoln, J. F. 1951. *What Makes Workers Work?* Cleveland, OH: The Lincoln Electric Company, pp. 3–4.

The ones who are crazy enough to think that they can change the world, are the ones who do.

—Steve Jobs

The Leader's Credo

10 points for warriors creating excellence in healthcare using gold standard management:

1. *We believe "the Customer is king."* It is a privilege to serve their cause. They trust us with their lives and the lives of their loved ones. They give us a supreme gift—the opportunity to do something meaningful with our lives. Our power is manifest by making it happen for them.

2. *Management is about winning.* Success is not simply trying hard, being sincere, and trudging off to another useless meeting. We will write down our goals, get others excited about them, make changes, and measure how we are doing. "A" Team members are passionate about this; "B" Team members do not work here.

3. *We are a family.* The golden rule always applies. If we expect people to stand by us, we must stand by them. We back each other, are kind to each other, and always approach each other with a mind to solve daily issues. We will be judged by the quality of our relationships.

4. *We are intolerant of mediocrity and bureaucratic thinking.* We reject all limited and "it will not work here" thinking. To do otherwise would negate our powers as people. Our inability to think differently is the only thing inherent in our situation that may cause us

to fail. We will always be positive minded. Leadership is all about edge, execution, and energy.

5. *We believe happiness in life is in direct proportion to our commitment to excellence.* Sloppy work, shoddy thinking, and half efforts have no part in what we do. The quality of our creative work matters and defines who we are. We will debate less. We will act more.

6. *We understand that leaders are not bosses, critics, or memo issuers.* They are teachers, servants, and appreciators. Leadership is not about us; it is about the team. We will work alongside the team, listen to their opinions, and change the organization to fit their needs. We will lead in only one way—by example.

7. *Our task is to find answers for many difficult problems.* Answers are abundant in our creative thinking as well as that of our team, patients, visitors, and physicians. Each day we will ask the golden question, "How can we do this better?"

8. *We will not wait for perfect answers.* We insist on partial, even small, improvements in the present. We expect to make mistakes in the process of making progress, but we will never make the mistake of defending the status quo.

9. *We embrace contrarianism.* We will not follow the herd. We will try what others have no courage to attempt. We will do what others say cannot be done.

10. *Failure in our task is not an option.* We will work with passion and persist. We will never give up. We will go the distance.

Additional Resources

For those adopting GSM, the following resources provide more information:

goldstandardmanagement.org
This nonprofit web site includes a resource library available to assist implementation of GSM practices. It also contains tactical plans for KRAs; course materials for management development; the MANSYS management system; guidance on how to conduct large-scale organizational transformation; and tools for organizatial diagnosis, cultural change, and performance enhancement.

Standards and Awards Organizations
Performance standards for healthcare organizations are changing. Many leaders use awards offered by the following groups as pacing targets for the organization, a tactic proven helpful in creating change:

* *The Leapfrog Group* (leapfroggroup.org) has an incentives program that provides financial incentives to hospitals meeting those standards.
* *Baldrige National Quality Program* (quality.nist.gov) provides certification, which many hospitals have attained, that drives change internally.

- *Governor's Award for Excellence, or the Governor's Award for Quality*, is provided by many states, often paralleling Baldrige criteria. Check to see if your state has one.
- *American Nurses Credential Center Magnet Certification* (nursecredentialing.org) is a way of distinguishing your organization as the employer of choice in the region.

There are other award programs sponsored by technical and professional groups. GSM thinking aggressively focuses the organization's "eyes on the prize." While prizes may be unimportant in themselves, what is vital is the creation of an organization that continuously thinks of itself as the best.

Intellectual Capital and Knowledge Management
The establishment of corporate universities in hospitals is an idea essential to all applied science businesses. Drive this development effort by adding a chief learning officer position. The next step is to create a management institute to assist with increasing professionalism for the organization's managers. Numerous free resources for management training materials and information exist that can be brought in-house. Resources include the following:

- Corporate University Xchange (corpu.com) is a free online resource.
- Numerous universities partner with organizations to provide online training. This can be a workable supplement under in-house coaching and assigned mentors.
- There are a number of good sites that contain free management development materials, including businessballs.com and managementhelp.org.

ABOUT THE AUTHORS

V. Clayton Sherman, Ed.D., is chairman of Management House, Inc., and a proponent of revolutionary management change approaches. He has worked with more than 1,000 hospitals and Fortune 500 companies. Dr. Sherman is the author of seven previous books, including Raising Standards in American Health Care and Creating the New American Hospital. His advocacy of benchmark management practices led to his induction as the charter member of the Studer Group's Healthcare Management Hall of Fame. Dr. Sherman serves as faculty for seminars on high-performance organizations and is the instructor of "Gold Standard Management," a program offered by the American College of Healthcare Executives (ACHE). His Uncommon Leader change program, which has helped clients win Governor's Gold Cup Awards, was chosen as semifinalist for USA Today's Quality Cup Award and won 3M's Innovations in Health Care Award. Dr. Sherman can be contacted at drclay@goldstandard management.org.

Stephanie G. Sherman is executive vice president of Management House, Inc. Her client list of more than 200 hospitals and health systems has allowed her to demonstrate the effectiveness of industry benchmarks. Ms. Sherman previously served as vice president of human resources at Mount Carmel Health System and global director of human resources for Rubbermaid. She is the author of five books, including Total Customer Satisfaction: A Comprehensive Approach for Healthcare Providers. Ms. Sherman can be reached at stephanie@goldstandard management.org.